Investigating ethical considerations and effective medicine across all demographics in the context of efficacy and safety. Rehabilitation's Resonance

Patient Recovery Through Holistic Therapies

Elowen Fairweather

Contents

1 Introduction to Holistic Rehabilitation

Holistic rehabilitation isn't simply about treating a broken bone or a debilitating illness; it's about addressing the whole person. This means considering the intricate interplay of physical, emotional, and social factors that influence a patient's recovery journey. We move beyond a purely biological focus, embracing a broader perspective that recognizes the individual's unique circumstances, beliefs, and support systems. It requires a collaborative approach, engaging not just medical professionals but also patients themselves, family members, and potentially complementary practitioners. This comprehensive model fosters a sense of empowerment and active participation in the healing process, resulting in improved outcomes and a better quality of life.

Unlike conventional models that might isolate symptoms or focus solely on physical limitations, a holistic approach seeks to understand the root cause of illness or injury. For example, chronic back pain might stem from poor posture, muscular imbalances, stress-related tension, or even underlying psychological factors. A holistic approach would investigate all these potential contributors, employing a range of interventions tailored to the individual's specific needs. This personalized treatment plan might include physiotherapy to address musculoskeletal issues, stress-reduction techniques like meditation or yoga to manage emotional factors, and ergonomic adjustments to improve work habits. The result is a much more comprehensive and effective approach to rehabilitation.

The benefits of this approach extend beyond simply regaining physical function. Holistic rehabilitation promotes emotional well-being, reducing stress and anxiety often associated with illness or injury. It cultivates a sense of self-efficacy and control, encouraging patients to actively participate in their recovery. Studies have shown that individuals receiving holistic care report increased satisfaction with their treatment, improved quality of life, and greater independence, all crucial aspects of successful rehabilitation. Furthermore, the holistic method often minimizes the reliance on medication, offering a less intrusive and potentially less harmful path to recovery. This is especially significant in situations where long-term medication use carries risks or side effects.

One key element of holistic rehabilitation is shared decision-making. It's not simply a matter of a medical professional dictating a treatment plan; it's about building a collaborative partnership between the healthcare provider and the patient. The patient's values, preferences, and goals are central to the treatment process. This partnership fosters trust, improves adherence to treatment plans, and ultimately leads to better outcomes. The patient's active participation in designing and implementing their recovery plan empowers them, reinforcing their sense of agency and accelerating their healing. This proactive involvement also reduces feelings of helplessness and fosters a more positive outlook on the rehabilitation journey.

The integration of complementary therapies adds another dimension to holistic rehabilitation. Techniques like acupuncture, massage, and mindfulness can complement conventional treatments, providing additional support for pain management, stress reduction, and emotional well-being. Evidence suggests that these therapies can be particularly beneficial when combined with more conventional approaches, providing a synergistic effect that enhances overall recovery. The effectiveness of these methods varies, and careful consideration is needed to ensure they are used appropriately, and their integration should always respect the patient's preferences and beliefs. It's imperative to always seek scientifically backed therapies.

The success of holistic rehabilitation hinges on a multidisciplinary team approach. Physical therapists, occupational therapists, psychologists, and other healthcare professionals work together, sharing their expertise to create a comprehensive treatment plan. This team approach helps address the complex needs of the patient, ensuring that all aspects of their well-being are considered. The collaborative environment fostered by this holistic approach encourages open communication and information sharing among the healthcare team, resulting in a more effective and well-rounded treatment plan. Furthermore, it promotes a more supportive and cohesive care environment for the patient.

However, there are challenges to implementing holistic rehabilitation approaches. One major obstacle is the integration of these methods into established healthcare systems, which are often structured around conventional, specialized models. Overcoming these structural barriers requires a shift in mindset, emphasizing the value and efficacy of holistic approaches. Furthermore, the increased time and resources often required for holistic assessment and treatment can present a practical challenge, particularly within resource-constrained healthcare settings. Addressing this challenge requires careful planning, resource allocation, and efficient workflow integration.

Despite the challenges, the potential benefits of holistic rehabilitation are undeniable. By embracing a more comprehensive and patient-centered approach, we can move beyond treating symptoms and focus on restoring the whole person to a state of health and well-being. It's a shift in paradigm that requires a commitment to collaborative practice, careful consideration of individual needs, and integration of diverse therapies. This forward-thinking approach not only enhances the effectiveness of rehabilitation but also fundamentally changes the patient experience, fostering empowerment, resilience, and overall well-being. The future of rehabilitation lies in a balanced approach that combines the strengths of conventional medicine with the holistic perspective, ultimately delivering optimal outcomes for patients across all demographics.

1.1 Defining Holistic Approach

A holistic approach to rehabilitation isn't simply about adding a few extra therapies to a standard treatment plan. It's a fundamental shift in perspective, a paradigm change that views the individual not as a collection of isolated symptoms, but as an interconnected whole. This means considering physical, emotional, mental, and social factors, all interwoven and influencing one another. A broken leg, for instance, might cause physical pain, but also lead to isolation, depression, and financial strain – all impacting the healing process. A holistic strategy addresses each of these intertwined elements, promoting a more complete and sustainable recovery.

Unlike a purely biomedical model focusing solely on the physiological aspects of illness and injury, a holistic approach embraces the complexity of human experience. It acknowledges that a patient's beliefs, cultural background, personal relationships, and overall lifestyle all play significant roles in their health and well-being. This understanding necessitates a collaborative relationship between the patient and the healthcare team, where shared decision-making is central to the treatment plan. The patient's voice becomes an integral part of the therapeutic process, guiding the direction and shaping the interventions.

Effective communication forms the bedrock of a successful holistic approach. It's not merely about conveying medical information; it's about establishing trust, fostering empathy, and creating a safe space for the patient to express their concerns and needs. Active listening, clear explanations, and the ability to tailor communication to the patient's understanding are crucial. This requires sensitivity to cultural nuances, language barriers, and individual learning styles. Ultimately, the goal is to empower the patient, making them an active participant in their own healing journey, rather than a passive recipient of treatment.

The integration of conventional medicine with complementary therapies presents unique opportunities within this framework. Physiotherapy and occupational therapy, for instance, offer valuable tools for restoring physical function, but their effectiveness can be enhanced when combined with techniques such as mindfulness or acupuncture. These complementary methods address the emotional and spiritual dimensions of health, often overlooked in purely biomedical approaches. A balanced strategy, drawing on the strengths of both conventional and complementary therapies, offers a more comprehensive and potentially more effective path towards recovery. It's essential to remember that rigorous scientific evaluation is necessary to ensure the efficacy and safety of all interventions, regardless of whether they fall under the conventional or complementary umbrella.

However, the implementation of a holistic approach is not without its challenges. The availability of qualified practitioners trained in both conventional and complementary modalities might be limited in some areas, impacting access to comprehensive care. Financial constraints can also pose a significant barrier, particularly if complementary therapies are not covered by insurance. Furthermore, the integration of diverse therapeutic approaches necessitates effective communication and collaboration between different healthcare professionals, requiring interdisciplinary teamwork and a shared understanding of holistic principles. Overcoming these challenges requires a multi-pronged approach, involving policy changes, professional training initiatives, and public awareness campaigns.

Finally, ethical considerations remain paramount. Informed consent, patient autonomy, and equitable access to care are fundamental principles that must guide the application of holistic approaches. Ensuring that patients fully understand their treatment options, have the freedom to make choices that align with their values, and are not excluded due to socioeconomic or other disparities, is not merely an ethical imperative but also crucial for maximizing the effectiveness of the approach. Rigorous monitoring of treatment efficacy and safety, coupled with a commitment to ongoing research, are vital for establishing evidence-based best practices and safeguarding patient well-being. Only through a meticulous attention to these considerations can the promise of a holistic approach to rehabilitation be realized, offering enhanced care, improved outcomes, and a more equitable healthcare system for all.

1.2 Benefits of Holistic Care

Holistic care offers a profound shift in perspective, moving beyond simply treating symptoms to addressing the interconnectedness of mind, body, and spirit. This integrated approach fosters a more comprehensive understanding of each patient's unique needs, creating a personalized treatment plan that considers their physical, emotional, and social well-being. For example, a patient recovering from a stroke might benefit not only from physical therapy to regain motor skills but also from counseling to address emotional trauma and support groups to combat isolation – elements often overlooked in purely conventional approaches.

Consider the impact of chronic pain. Conventional medicine frequently focuses on pain management through medication, which, while effective in some cases, may have undesirable side effects and fail to address the underlying causes. A holistic approach, however, might incorporate techniques like acupuncture, mindfulness meditation, or physical therapy to address the root of the problem, fostering self-management skills that reduce reliance on medication and promote lasting relief. This integrated approach also empowers the patient to actively participate in their recovery process, enhancing engagement and boosting the overall effectiveness of the treatment.

The benefits extend beyond individual healing. Studies suggest that holistic care can lead to decreased healthcare costs in the long run. By addressing preventative health and wellness, reducing the frequency of acute episodes, and enhancing self-management capabilities, individuals may experience less frequent hospitalizations and reduce their overall healthcare burden. This economic advantage is further compounded by improved quality of life, which allows patients to maintain greater independence and contribute actively to society—a significant social and economic benefit for communities.

However, the integration of holistic practices also presents challenges. A fundamental obstacle is the lack of standardized protocols and outcome measures for many complementary therapies. This makes it challenging to establish evidence-based efficacy and compare their effectiveness against conventional approaches. Moreover, the reimbursement landscape for holistic therapies often lacks the clarity and consistency found in conventional medicine, creating barriers to access and potentially compromising the financial viability of these integrated approaches for practitioners.

Overcoming these obstacles requires collaboration between healthcare professionals from various disciplines. Physicians, therapists, and practitioners of complementary therapies need to share knowledge and develop effective communication strategies to integrate their perspectives seamlessly. This unified approach is not about replacing conventional medicine but rather about creating a supportive ecosystem where conventional and holistic practices complement each other, creating synergy for better patient outcomes.

Furthermore, the ethical dimensions of holistic care are significant. Patients need to be fully informed about the benefits and limitations of various therapies, including the lack of definitive scientific evidence for some practices. Ensuring informed consent is crucial, as is maintaining confidentiality and respecting patient autonomy throughout the process. Open communication and a shared decision-making model between healthcare providers and patients is paramount to ethically sound holistic care.

Ultimately, the integration of holistic care into mainstream healthcare reflects a profound shift towards patient-centered care. The ability to address the whole person – encompassing physical, emotional, social, and spiritual aspects – has the potential to profoundly improve the patient journey, fostering healthier outcomes and a more fulfilling life. It signifies a movement beyond merely treating illness to nurturing wellness. The journey towards this integration, however, necessitates addressing the challenges of standardization, reimbursement, and ethical considerations, requiring collaborative efforts across disciplines and a commitment to evidence-based practice. The result, however, promises a future of healthcare that is more humane, effective, and holistic.

2 Ethical Considerations in Healthcare

Informed consent is paramount. It's not just about signing a form; it's about ensuring patients truly understand their treatment options, the potential risks and benefits, and feel empowered to make choices aligned with their values and beliefs. This requires clear, compassionate communication tailored to the individual's comprehension level, cultural background, and emotional state. Ignoring this fundamental principle risks undermining patient autonomy and eroding trust in the healthcare system. A thorough explanation, using plain language and avoiding medical jargon, is vital. Furthermore, documenting this process meticulously safeguards against misunderstandings and potential legal challenges. The process should be interactive, encouraging questions and ensuring the patient feels comfortable expressing any concerns. Ultimately, informed consent fosters a collaborative relationship, empowering patients to actively participate in their own care.

Equity in healthcare demands that every individual, regardless of their socioeconomic status, race, ethnicity, gender, or geographic location, has equal access to high-quality rehabilitation services. Disparities persist, often rooted in systemic inequalities such as limited access to healthcare insurance, geographic isolation,

or cultural biases within the healthcare system itself. Addressing these requires a multifaceted approach, including policy changes to improve insurance coverage, targeted outreach programs to underserved communities, and cultural competency training for healthcare professionals. Beyond simple access, true equity means ensuring culturally appropriate care, meaning services are delivered in ways that respect and accommodate individual cultural beliefs and practices. It requires recognizing and addressing potential implicit biases that may influence the delivery of care. Ultimately, this requires ongoing reflection, education, and commitment from both policymakers and healthcare professionals.
Maintaining patient confidentiality and privacy is not merely a legal obligation; it's a cornerstone of ethical healthcare practice. The trust between a patient and their healthcare provider is built upon the assurance that personal information will be protected. This includes medical history, diagnoses, treatment plans, and any other sensitive personal data. Breaches of confidentiality can have devastating consequences, causing emotional harm and damaging the patient-provider relationship. Healthcare professionals must rigorously adhere to legal regulations such as HIPAA in the United States, or equivalent legislation in other countries, and maintain secure record-keeping systems. Furthermore, the ethical responsibility extends beyond legal mandates, demanding discretion and thoughtful consideration of the potential impact of information sharing at every juncture. Openly discussing privacy policies and obtaining consent for information sharing are crucial steps to maintaining trust and respecting patient autonomy.

The intersection of culture and healthcare is profoundly significant. Cultural beliefs and practices can profoundly influence a patient's understanding of illness, their choices regarding treatment, and their overall adherence to a rehabilitation plan. For instance, some cultures may prefer traditional healing methods alongside conventional care, while others might hold beliefs that affect their willingness to accept specific medical interventions. A culturally competent approach necessitates healthcare providers develop sensitivity and understanding of different cultural perspectives on health, illness, and healing. This involves ongoing learning, respectful communication, and the willingness to adapt treatment approaches to better meet the needs and preferences of diverse patients. Ignoring cultural factors can lead to miscommunication, misunderstandings, and ultimately, ineffective or even harmful treatment. Respecting diverse perspectives is not just good ethics; it's vital for achieving effective and equitable healthcare. Effective communication is pivotal, and sometimes necessitates using interpreters or culturally sensitive resources.

The ethical implications of using technology in healthcare are far-reaching. Technological advancements offer unprecedented opportunities to improve diagnosis, treatment, and rehabilitation outcomes. However, they also raise ethical questions concerning data privacy, algorithmic bias, and the potential for widening existing health disparities. Ensuring equitable access to innovative technologies is crucial, preventing a scenario where only certain segments of the population benefit. Furthermore, careful consideration must be given to the potential for algorithmic bias, as algorithms trained on biased data may perpetuate and even exacerbate existing health inequalities. Transparency and accountability in the development and use of health technologies are also vital to build trust and ensure responsible innovation. Healthcare professionals and policymakers must actively engage in discussions concerning the ethical implications of these technologies to mitigate risks and maximize their potential benefits for all.

2.1 Informed Consent & Autonomy

Informed consent is the cornerstone of ethical healthcare practice. It's not merely a signature on a form; it's a dynamic process built on mutual understanding and respect. True informed consent requires the patient to possess a clear comprehension of their condition, the proposed treatment options, including potential risks and benefits, and the alternatives available, if any. This understanding must be achieved in a way that respects the patient's individual capabilities and communication style. Failure to provide sufficient information, or using jargon that obscures understanding, is a breach of ethical obligations and might lead to legal ramifications. Clinicians should tailor their explanations to the patient's comprehension level, actively checking for understanding throughout the process and answering questions with patience and clarity. The patient's right to refuse treatment, even if it seems medically beneficial, remains paramount. This underscores the vital importance of open and honest communication.

Autonomy, the right to self-determination, is intrinsically linked to informed consent. It recognizes the patient's capacity for self-governance and their right to make choices about their own body and healthcare. This implies respecting the patient's decisions, even if those choices differ from what healthcare professionals might advise. However, autonomy isn't absolute. If a patient lacks the capacity to make informed decisions, whether due to cognitive impairment, mental illness, or other factors, a surrogate decision-maker may be necessary. Identifying this incapacity requires careful assessment and should always involve collaboration with the patient's family or legal representatives, if applicable. Ethical considerations dictate that these surrogates should act in the patient's best interests, mirroring the choices the patient would likely make if they possessed the capacity.

The concept of capacity itself is nuanced and context-dependent. It's not a binary state of either competent or incompetent; rather, it exists on a spectrum. A patient might have capacity to decide about some aspects of their treatment but lack it regarding others. For instance, a patient might understand the nature of their illness and the proposed surgery but lack the capacity to comprehend the potential long-term complications. In such situations, a collaborative approach involving careful assessment by healthcare professionals, perhaps including specialists in geriatrics or neuropsychology, becomes crucial. The focus should always remain on supporting the patient's autonomy to the greatest extent possible while safeguarding their well-being. A multidisciplinary team approach, which includes input from family members when appropriate, can help create a comprehensive understanding of the patient's best interests and capacities.

Furthermore, cultural factors significantly influence the understanding and application of informed consent and autonomy. In some cultures, family involvement in healthcare decisions is deeply ingrained, while in others, individual autonomy takes precedence. Healthcare professionals must be sensitive to these cultural nuances, ensuring that the process of obtaining informed consent is culturally appropriate and respects the patient's values and beliefs. This requires a deep understanding of the cultural background of the patient, possibly involving culturally sensitive interpreters or seeking advice from cultural experts. It's not merely about providing translated materials; it's about adapting the communication style and approach to resonate with the patient's cultural context. Failing to account for these cultural factors could lead to misunderstandings, mistrust, and compromised healthcare outcomes.

Transparency and open communication are pivotal throughout the rehabilitation process. This necessitates creating an environment where patients feel comfortable asking questions and expressing concerns. Healthcare professionals should proactively address potential anxieties related to treatment, recovery timelines, and potential complications. Regular updates on the patient's progress, involving them in the decision-making process about their treatment plan adjustments, fosters trust and reinforces the principles of informed consent and patient autonomy. This collaborative approach not only improves patient compliance and satisfaction but also leads to better outcomes overall. Regular feedback loops, through documented progress reports and informal conversations, ensure that the patient feels heard and actively involved in their journey to recovery, thereby strengthening their sense of agency and control over their health. This collaborative approach empowers patients and fosters a healing environment built upon mutual trust and respect.

2.2 Equity and Access to Care

Healthcare disparities significantly impact access to rehabilitation services. Socioeconomic status, geographical location, and insurance coverage are major barriers. Many individuals from low-income backgrounds lack adequate transportation to reach rehabilitation facilities, facing further hurdles with inflexible appointment scheduling that clashes with work commitments or childcare responsibilities. This results in delayed or absent access to crucial therapies, impeding recovery and potentially exacerbating existing health conditions. The consequences can be devastating, leading to prolonged disability, diminished quality of life, and increased healthcare costs in the long run. Addressing these systemic inequalities demands a multi-pronged approach, incorporating policy changes and community-based initiatives.

Addressing the challenge of equitable access requires a proactive strategy encompassing several interconnected elements. Firstly, policy adjustments are crucial. Expanding healthcare coverage to include comprehensive rehabilitation services is paramount. Governmental support and funding should target underserved communities, ensuring affordability and accessibility for all. This includes funding transportation assistance, flexible scheduling options, and culturally competent rehabilitation programs that address the specific needs of diverse patient populations. The creation of mobile rehabilitation units in underserved areas could also prove highly impactful.

Secondly, fostering collaboration between healthcare providers and community organizations proves vital. Establishing partnerships with local community centers, churches, and non-profit organizations can assist in disseminating information about available rehabilitation services. These partnerships can also help bridge the cultural gap, providing outreach services tailored to the specific linguistic and cultural needs of individual communities. This community-based approach should prioritize patient education and engagement, empowering individuals to advocate for their healthcare needs effectively. Training programs for community health workers could further enhance outreach and support systems.

Thirdly, a commitment to data collection and analysis is imperative to understand and address the root causes of disparities. Systematic tracking of patient demographics, access to care, and treatment outcomes is essential. This allows for the identification of trends and patterns, informing the development of targeted interventions to rectify existing inequalities. Regular audits of healthcare systems should be conducted, focusing on fairness and equity in resource allocation and service provision. Openly sharing findings with relevant stakeholders facilitates improvements in accessibility and quality of care.

Furthermore, innovative financing models may also enhance equity. Exploring options such as pay-for-performance models and value-based care systems can incentivize healthcare providers to focus on improving access and outcomes for all patients, regardless of their background. These models could reward providers who effectively reach underserved populations and achieve positive patient outcomes, motivating a more equitable distribution of resources and services. The integration of telehealth technologies can also expand access to care for individuals in remote or underserved areas, overcoming geographical barriers and ensuring timely intervention.

Beyond systemic changes, individual healthcare professionals also hold a pivotal role in fostering equity. Practitioners should actively seek to understand and address individual patient circumstances, demonstrating empathy and cultural sensitivity in their interactions. This involves taking the time to discuss potential barriers to care openly, offering solutions where possible. Providing culturally appropriate materials and education, and ensuring linguistic access through translation services, further enhances inclusivity and engagement. A commitment to ongoing professional development in cultural competence and health equity further strengthens the ability of healthcare practitioners to meet the needs of diverse patient populations. It's a continuous process requiring ongoing reflection and adaptation.

Finally, we must acknowledge the complex interplay of factors influencing access to care. Addressing these requires a nuanced and holistic strategy, combining policy reform, community engagement, data-driven interventions, and a fundamental shift in the way healthcare professionals approach patient care. Promoting health equity isn't simply a matter of providing services; it demands a commitment to dismantling systemic barriers, fostering inclusivity, and ensuring that every individual has the opportunity to achieve optimal health and well-being, regardless of their background. This continuous commitment to equitable access is not just an ethical imperative; it's essential for building a truly resilient and just healthcare system.

2.3 Confidentiality & Privacy

Maintaining patient confidentiality and privacy is paramount in rehabilitation, a cornerstone of ethical healthcare practice. Breaches of confidentiality can severely damage the therapeutic relationship, undermining trust and hindering the recovery process. Legal repercussions, including lawsuits and professional sanctions, are also significant concerns. Therefore, robust protocols must be implemented and rigorously followed.

The Health Insurance Portability and Accountability Act (HIPAA) in the United States, and similar legislation in other countries, provides a framework for protecting patient health information. Understanding these regulations is crucial for healthcare professionals. Beyond legal compliance, however, upholding confidentiality is a moral imperative, reflecting a commitment to patient well-being and fostering a safe environment for vulnerable individuals to share their experiences.

Effective communication is key. Clearly explaining to patients how their information will be used and protected fosters transparency and builds trust. This includes explaining the limits of confidentiality, such as mandatory reporting requirements for child abuse or threats of self-harm. Obtaining informed consent for the release of information to other healthcare providers or insurers is also vital. This process should be documented meticulously, ensuring accuracy and providing a clear audit trail.

Technological advancements present both opportunities and challenges. Electronic health records (EHRs) offer significant improvements in efficiency and data management, but they also increase the risk of data breaches. Robust cybersecurity measures, including secure password management, firewalls, and regular software updates, are essential to protect sensitive information. Staff training on data security protocols is equally critical, ensuring that all personnel understand their responsibilities and adhere to established guidelines.

Beyond digital security, physical security measures are also necessary. Access to patient files should be restricted to authorized personnel only, with appropriate security measures in place. Physical files should be stored securely, locked away when not in use. Shredding or secure disposal of outdated or sensitive documents is essential to prevent unauthorized access.

Maintaining patient privacy extends beyond information management. Respectful communication and a commitment to non-judgmental care are vital aspects of privacy protection. Conversations about sensitive topics should occur in private settings, ensuring that patients feel comfortable and secure sharing their concerns. Moreover, understanding and respecting cultural differences regarding disclosure and privacy is essential in providing culturally sensitive care.

The use of patient information for research purposes requires careful consideration of ethical implications. Anonymization and de-identification techniques are crucial for safeguarding patient identities. Obtaining informed consent for research participation, including the clear explanation of data usage and storage protocols, is essential. Furthermore, adherence to institutional review board (IRB) guidelines and regulations ensures ethical compliance.

Finally, developing a culture of confidentiality and privacy within the rehabilitation setting is crucial. Regular staff training, clear policies and procedures, and effective communication are all essential components. Addressing breaches of confidentiality swiftly and transparently helps build trust and reinforce the importance of these ethical principles. A culture that values and prioritizes patient confidentiality and privacy fosters a healing environment where patients feel empowered and secure in their treatment. These actions demonstrate professionalism and ethical commitment and directly contribute to optimal patient outcomes and long-term rehabilitation success. Ultimately, the protection of patient confidentiality and privacy is not merely a legal requirement; it's a moral imperative that underpins the foundation of trust in the therapeutic relationship, directly impacting the efficacy and safety of holistic care. Consistently upholding these standards ensures a higher quality of care and respect for human dignity.

3 Effective Medication Across Demographics

Geriatric patients often metabolize medications differently than younger adults. Their slower metabolic rates can lead to increased drug accumulation, potentially causing adverse effects. Conversely, reduced liver and kidney function can result in lower drug concentrations, lessening the therapeutic effect. Therefore, careful dose adjustments are crucial, frequently requiring lower initial doses and more vigilant monitoring for both efficacy and side effects. Understanding these pharmacokinetic variations is paramount for safe and effective treatment in older populations. This necessitates a nuanced approach to medication management, tailoring treatments to individual physiological characteristics rather than adhering rigidly to standard dosage guidelines. Failure to consider these age-related differences can lead to serious complications, underscoring the importance of comprehensive geriatric assessment prior to prescribing any medication. This individualized approach should also include careful consideration of potential drug interactions, as polypharmacy—the simultaneous use of multiple medications—is common in older adults and increases the risk of adverse reactions. Detailed patient history, including current medications, allergies and pre-existing conditions, is absolutely essential for minimizing these risks.

Cultural beliefs significantly influence medication adherence and treatment choices. Some cultures may favor traditional medicine, while others may distrust Western pharmaceuticals. These beliefs can affect a patient's willingness to comply with prescribed regimens or even their acceptance of a diagnosis itself. For example, a patient's cultural background might influence their perception of pain, impacting their response to analgesic medications. Similarly, cultural norms surrounding health communication can influence how effectively patients communicate their symptoms and treatment preferences to healthcare providers. Effective communication is therefore essential for ensuring culturally sensitive care and achieving optimal treatment outcomes. It's crucial to avoid imposing culturally biased assumptions; instead, healthcare providers must actively listen to patients' concerns and beliefs, ensuring a partnership built on mutual respect and understanding. Bridging cultural divides requires sensitivity, patience, and a genuine effort to understand the patient's perspective. This involves not just adapting language but adapting the entire therapeutic approach to better align with the patient's cultural framework. Understanding a patient's cultural background goes beyond simply knowing their ethnicity; it's about understanding their beliefs about illness, health, and treatment, acknowledging their personal values and preferences.

Addressing health disparities among different demographic groups necessitates a proactive approach. Socioeconomic factors, such as access to healthcare and health insurance, significantly impact a person's ability to afford and obtain necessary medications. Geographical location plays a crucial role, with rural populations often facing greater challenges in accessing specialists and pharmacies. Lack of adequate health literacy further complicates the situation, as patients may struggle to understand instructions or communicate their needs effectively. To combat this, comprehensive healthcare initiatives must strive to address the underlying social determinants of health. This may include supporting community-based health programs, expanding access to affordable insurance and medications, and investing in health literacy programs tailored to diverse populations. Addressing these disparities requires understanding the intersectional nature of social inequities and implementing solutions that address systemic issues, not just individual cases. This commitment to health equity goes beyond simple provision of resources; it involves fundamentally rethinking how healthcare is structured and delivered. The goal is to create a system where all individuals, regardless of their social background, have equal opportunities to achieve optimal health and well-being.

Effective medication management extends beyond merely prescribing the correct drug. Patient education is key to ensure adherence and reduce the risk of medication errors. Providing clear, concise instructions, explaining potential side effects, and encouraging open communication between patient and provider are crucial steps. It's vital to tailor the education approach to the individual's level of health literacy, ensuring they fully understand their medication regimen. Empowering patients to actively participate in their healthcare journey enhances their compliance and fosters a sense of ownership over their treatment plan. By educating patients about their medications, healthcare providers are building trust and improving overall healthcare outcomes. It's about facilitating understanding—not just handing over prescriptions. Furthermore, follow-up appointments are essential to monitor progress, address any concerns, and make adjustments as needed. Regular check-ups allow providers to assess the efficacy of the medication and make necessary changes, thus maximizing treatment benefit and minimizing potential risks. This ongoing monitoring ensures that the treatment remains effective and safe, adapting to the individual's changing needs and circumstances.

3.1 Age-Related Medication Differences

Pharmacokinetic and pharmacodynamic changes associated with aging significantly impact medication efficacy and safety. Older adults often exhibit decreased renal and hepatic function, leading to slower drug metabolism and excretion. This results in prolonged drug half-lives, increasing the risk of drug accumulation and adverse effects, even at standard dosages. Consequently, careful dose adjustments are crucial, often requiring lower initial doses and close monitoring for adverse events. We must remember that this isn't a simple matter of reducing dosages across the board; individual patient factors such as comorbidities, polypharmacy, and nutritional status further complicate medication management in the elderly.

Polypharmacy, the concurrent use of multiple medications, is particularly prevalent among older adults and presents a unique challenge. The increased risk of drug interactions, both synergistic and antagonistic, significantly complicates treatment and necessitates careful medication reconciliation. This process involves a thorough review of all medications a patient is taking—prescription, over-the-counter, and herbal remedies—to identify potential interactions and optimize the medication regimen. Healthcare providers need to proactively identify and address potential drug-drug interactions, and patient education on the importance of disclosing all medications is paramount.

Beyond physiological changes, cognitive decline can impact medication adherence in older adults. Difficulties with memory, understanding instructions, or managing multiple medications can lead to missed doses, incorrect dosage administration, or altogether abandoning prescribed treatment plans. Simple strategies, such as pill organizers, clearly labeled medications, and regular communication with healthcare professionals, can significantly improve adherence rates. In cases of severe cognitive impairment, family involvement and caregiver support may be essential. Remembering that the goal isn't simply dispensing medication, but ensuring patients understand and actively participate in their treatment plan is vital for effective outcomes.

The use of medications with a narrow therapeutic index, where the difference between therapeutic and toxic doses is small, requires heightened caution in older adults. Drugs such as digoxin and warfarin demand meticulous monitoring of serum drug levels and careful titration to avoid toxicity. Regular blood tests are frequently necessary to ensure safe and effective treatment, and it's not only about blood tests; clinicians should work closely with pharmacists and specialists to tailor treatment plans specifically to each patient's unique circumstances. Furthermore, geriatric specialists possess the expertise to navigate the complexities of medication management in older populations, offering crucial insights into safe and effective medication choices and dose adjustments.

Beyond the purely physiological, geriatric syndromes, such as frailty, cognitive impairment, and falls, commonly affect older individuals and often necessitate medication adjustments. For instance, medications with anticholinergic effects, which can cause drowsiness, confusion, and constipation, may exacerbate cognitive decline and increase the risk of falls. A comprehensive geriatric assessment, including a review of medications, can identify potential risk factors and guide medication choices to minimize such complications. This requires not just expertise in geriatrics but a holistic view of the patient's overall health and functional abilities. Careful consideration of the risks and benefits of each medication is necessary, considering its impact on various aspects of the patient's health and daily life.

The ethical implications of prescribing medications to older adults should never be ignored. Shared decision-making, involving the patient and their family in the treatment process, is essential to ensure that treatment aligns with their values and preferences. Respecting patient autonomy is paramount, even when cognitive function is impaired, and the use of advance care planning tools can help guide medication choices in line with the patient's long-term goals. This necessitates that healthcare professionals engage in sensitive and respectful communication, ensuring patients feel heard and empowered to participate in their own care. Open and honest communication with patients and their families is key to ensuring ethical considerations are paramount in medication decisions. Finally, continuous monitoring and evaluation of medication efficacy and safety in older adults are vital. Regular review of medication lists, assessment of adverse effects, and adjustments to dosage as needed are crucial to ensure optimal treatment outcomes. This ongoing process of monitoring and adjustment highlights the importance of longitudinal care, rather than one-off interventions. The patient's overall health and well-being should always be the focus of medication decisions, and regular follow-up care is essential for identifying any emerging problems and adjusting the treatment plan as needed. The focus remains on maximizing benefits while minimizing potential harms, providing personalized care tailored to the unique needs and vulnerabilities of each individual.

3.2 Cultural Considerations in Treatment

Understanding a patient's cultural background is paramount to effective treatment. It's not simply about acknowledging their ethnicity; it's about deeply understanding their beliefs, values, and practices concerning health, illness, and healing. These deeply ingrained perspectives significantly influence how they perceive their condition, their willingness to participate in treatment, and their overall recovery journey. Ignoring these cultural nuances can lead to misunderstandings, treatment resistance, and ultimately, suboptimal outcomes. We must move beyond superficial understanding.

Effective communication is the cornerstone of culturally sensitive care. This goes beyond simply translating medical jargon into their native language. It demands active listening, empathy, and a genuine effort to understand their perspective, even if it differs vastly from our own. For example, a patient's reluctance to disclose certain symptoms might stem from cultural norms surrounding modesty or family honor. Ignoring this could lead to a misdiagnosis and hinder their recovery. Building rapport requires patience, cultural humility, and a willingness to learn. Effective communication may require engaging family members or community leaders in the process, as their input can be invaluable. We should not underestimate the significance of this stage.

Cultural beliefs about illness can profoundly shape a patient's approach to treatment. Some cultures attribute illness to supernatural causes, while others focus on the imbalance of bodily energies. These beliefs aren't simply irrational; they're integral to the patient's understanding of their health and well-being. A treatment plan that dismisses these beliefs risks alienating the patient and undermining their trust. A more effective strategy might involve integrating culturally acceptable healing practices into the treatment plan, whenever possible, without compromising medical integrity. This sensitive approach acknowledges the patient's beliefs while maintaining a scientific foundation for care. A collaborative approach, combining traditional medicine with the patient's cultural beliefs, may foster more effective treatment and increase adherence.

Furthermore, cultural differences extend to communication styles and family dynamics. In some cultures, direct confrontation is avoided, while in others, open and assertive communication is preferred. Understanding these nuances is crucial in establishing a therapeutic alliance. The involvement of family members in decision-making can vary widely across cultures, influencing the informed consent process and treatment adherence. Recognizing these differences will help us tailor our communication and approach to ensure effective collaboration and respect for the patient's cultural values. Failure to do so can lead to conflicts and create barriers to effective treatment. Sensitivity and cultural awareness are necessary to navigate these complex dynamics.

Access to healthcare services is often influenced by cultural factors. Language barriers, cultural misunderstandings about healthcare systems, and the lack of culturally competent healthcare providers can all impede access. Transportation issues and financial constraints are also significantly affected by sociocultural influences. We must address these systemic barriers proactively, advocating for improved access, training culturally sensitive healthcare providers, and building bridges between healthcare systems and diverse communities. A proactive approach, addressing these systemic issues, will enhance the likelihood of treatment success.

Finally, cultural influences on medication adherence are undeniable. Factors such as beliefs about the effectiveness of medication, trust in healthcare providers, and the affordability of prescription drugs can all impact medication adherence. Furthermore, cultural beliefs about herbal remedies or alternative medicine might lead to a patient choosing to forgo prescribed medication. This is not necessarily a sign of non-compliance but rather a reflection of their beliefs and cultural preferences. We must work collaboratively with patients, understanding these beliefs to help them understand the effectiveness and safety of the prescribed medications. Education and respectful communication will always increase the likelihood of effective cooperation. A holistic approach incorporating patient beliefs can significantly enhance treatment adherence.

4 Efficacy and Safety in Treatment

Precise measurement of treatment efficacy is paramount. We must move beyond subjective assessments and embrace rigorous, quantifiable metrics. This might involve tracking functional improvements using standardized scales like the Functional Independence Measure (FIM) or the Barthel Index, carefully monitoring physiological indicators relevant to the specific condition, and consistently documenting patient-reported outcome measures (PROMs) to capture their lived experience of recovery. The data collected should be meticulously recorded, ensuring accuracy and minimizing bias. Statistical analysis, using appropriate methods, is crucial for drawing valid conclusions about the effectiveness of the interventions. Finally, regular audits and quality control measures are necessary to maintain high standards and ensure the reliability of our findings.

Ensuring patient safety is an ethical imperative and fundamental to effective rehabilitation. A comprehensive safety protocol, integrated into every aspect of treatment, is essential. This encompasses meticulous risk assessment, identifying potential hazards specific to the individual patient and their condition. Clear communication with patients, including detailed explanations of procedures and potential risks, is crucial to fostering trust and informed consent. Regular monitoring of vital signs and careful observation for any adverse reactions are fundamental. The implementation of appropriate safety measures, such as fall prevention strategies and modifications to the environment, reduces potential risks. Prompt response to any identified safety concerns and thorough documentation of all safety-related incidents are non-negotiable components of a safe rehabilitation environment.

Adverse effects, unfortunately, are an inherent part of many treatments. Early identification is key, requiring vigilant monitoring of patients for any unusual symptoms or changes in their condition. A robust system for reporting and documenting adverse events is essential, allowing for timely intervention and analysis. Effective management of adverse effects requires a multi-faceted approach, ranging from dose adjustment and medication changes to supportive care measures aimed at alleviating symptoms and improving patient comfort. Collaboration amongst healthcare professionals is crucial, ensuring coordinated care and optimizing outcomes. Thorough documentation of adverse events, their management, and the patient's response is not only ethically responsible but essential for continuous quality improvement and future research.

Data analysis and interpretation are critical for guiding future research and optimizing treatment protocols. The collected data, whether from clinical trials or routine practice, must be analyzed using appropriate statistical methods to determine the significance of our findings. Understanding the limitations of the data is as important as the results themselves. This requires a clear understanding of statistical concepts and the ability to interpret complex data sets. Moreover, the results must be translated into practical recommendations for improving clinical practice. Regular review of data, alongside feedback from patients and clinicians, ensures the continuous improvement and refinement of treatment strategies.

Future research in holistic rehabilitation needs to prioritize several key areas. We must move towards more rigorous research designs, such as randomized controlled trials, to provide stronger evidence for the efficacy of specific holistic therapies. This will involve careful consideration of study design, sampling methods, and statistical analysis. Furthermore, there's a need for longitudinal studies to track patient outcomes over the long term, gaining a more comprehensive understanding of the sustained effects of various interventions. This research must also address the issue of equitable access, ensuring that our findings benefit all populations, irrespective of socioeconomic status or geographical location. Finally, exploring the biological mechanisms underlying the effectiveness of holistic therapies will deepen our understanding and pave the way for more targeted interventions.

4.1 Measuring Treatment Efficacy

Establishing objective measures of treatment efficacy in rehabilitation requires a multifaceted approach, moving beyond simple symptom reduction. We need to consider functional improvements, quality of life enhancements, and the patient's subjective experience. A purely quantitative approach, relying solely on numerical data, overlooks the nuanced reality of patient recovery. For example, a patient might show a slight decrease in pain scores, but still report significant limitations in daily activities. This highlights the need for a more holistic assessment incorporating qualitative data.

Effective measurement necessitates a baseline assessment before treatment commences. This involves documenting the patient's current functional abilities, pain levels, and overall well-being using standardized tools, including validated questionnaires and physical performance tests. This detailed baseline provides a benchmark against which subsequent progress can be reliably measured. Consider, for example, the use of the Functional Independence Measure (FIM) or the Oswestry Disability Index (ODI), depending on the specific condition and treatment goals. The chosen instrument must be appropriate for the patient's condition and cognitive abilities. It's crucial to ensure consistent and accurate data collection throughout the treatment process.

Beyond standardized tools, incorporating regular qualitative data is essential. This involves ongoing conversations with the patient, actively listening to their experiences, understanding their challenges, and tracking their perceptions of improvement. This qualitative information adds depth and context to the quantitative data, providing a richer understanding of the treatment's impact on the individual's life. Open-ended questions, focused on the patient's daily activities and overall satisfaction, can reveal invaluable insights that purely numerical measures might miss. Remember, the patient's voice holds tremendous weight in evaluating treatment efficacy.

The timing and frequency of assessments are crucial. Regular evaluations allow for prompt identification of treatment response or lack thereof. This allows for necessary adjustments to the treatment plan, maximizing its effectiveness and optimizing patient outcomes. The frequency of assessment will naturally vary depending on the patient's condition and treatment modality. However, consistent monitoring, perhaps weekly or bi-weekly initially, ensures a responsive treatment approach. This enables early detection of potential complications or adverse effects, allowing for timely interventions.

Data analysis should go beyond simple comparisons of pre\item and post-treatment scores. It should also involve exploring correlations between various measures, identifying factors influencing treatment outcomes, and investigating potential confounding variables. Analyzing data within the context of individual patient characteristics— age, pre-existing conditions, adherence to the treatment plan, and lifestyle factors—is critical to discerning genuine treatment effects. This multifaceted approach requires a blend of statistical methods and clinical judgment to accurately interpret the results and draw meaningful conclusions.

Moreover, the measurement of treatment efficacy must account for the long-term impact of the intervention. This means following up with patients over an extended period, assessing the durability of treatment effects and identifying potential long-term benefits or complications. Regular follow-up assessments can provide invaluable information about the sustained impact of the therapy, revealing its true effectiveness over time. Longitudinal studies are invaluable for assessing true treatment success and durability and informing future treatment strategies and protocols.

Finally, transparency and ethical considerations are paramount. Patients must be fully informed about the methods used to evaluate their treatment progress and how the data will be used. Respect for patient autonomy is crucial, and their participation in the process should be voluntary and informed. Data must be handled ethically and confidentially, adhering to all relevant regulations and guidelines. This fosters trust between the healthcare provider and patient, crucial for effective and successful treatment. Only through a holistic, ethical approach can we truly measure the efficacy of interventions and ensure optimal patient care.

4.2 Ensuring Patient Safety

Minimizing risks is paramount in any healthcare setting, especially within the context of rehabilitation. A proactive approach to patient safety encompasses multiple layers, from meticulous record-keeping to comprehensive staff training. Thorough documentation of each patient's medical history, treatment plan, and progress notes forms a critical foundation for safety. This detailed record allows for informed decision-making and efficient communication among the healthcare team, preventing errors stemming from incomplete or missing information. Regular review of these records is essential, serving as an opportunity to identify potential issues and proactively adjust the treatment plan as needed. Furthermore, meticulous documentation provides legal protection and facilitates continuity of care should a patient transfer to another facility. A comprehensive record allows a new team to quickly understand the patient's history, reducing the risk of errors.

Effective communication is the lifeblood of a safe rehabilitation environment. Clear and concise communication between healthcare professionals, patients, and their families is vital. This necessitates the use of plain language, avoiding medical jargon that may confuse or intimidate patients. Active listening, ensuring mutual understanding, and providing opportunities for patients and families to ask questions should be prioritized. Establishing a safe space where patients feel comfortable expressing concerns is essential. Regular team meetings offer a forum to discuss individual patient cases, share observations, and collaboratively develop strategies to address potential risks. This collaborative approach fosters a culture of shared responsibility for patient well-being.

Implementing standardized protocols and procedures across all aspects of patient care is crucial for minimizing errors and enhancing safety. These protocols should cover everything from medication administration and equipment usage to emergency response procedures. Adherence to established guidelines minimizes variability in treatment, reducing the likelihood of mistakes. Regular audits and quality control measures are critical to ensure continued compliance with these protocols. This ongoing evaluation process identifies areas for improvement and ensures that protocols remain up-to-date with current best practices, enhancing patient safety continually. A system of regular checks and balances is essential.

Regular safety inspections of equipment and the environment are crucial. Malfunctioning equipment can lead to serious injuries, while hazardous environments increase the risk of falls or accidents. Therefore, a preventative maintenance schedule for all equipment is essential, coupled with regular environmental safety checks. This process involves regularly inspecting the facility for potential hazards, such as loose wires, uneven flooring, or insufficient lighting. Any identified hazards need immediate remediation to ensure a safe environment for both patients and staff. The commitment to safety should be clearly communicated to all staff, establishing a shared responsibility to report any potential safety concerns promptly.

Patient education is a cornerstone of effective rehabilitation and a critical component of ensuring patient safety. Empowering patients with the knowledge and skills to participate actively in their recovery enhances their sense of control and reduces the risk of errors. Patients should be educated about their treatment plan, potential side effects of medications, and any necessary precautions. This education promotes adherence to the treatment plan, minimizing the potential for adverse events. Encouraging open dialogue and actively addressing any questions or concerns contribute to a strong patient-provider relationship, fostering trust and cooperation.

Finally, a strong emphasis on continuous learning and professional development for all staff members is crucial. Healthcare professionals must keep abreast of the latest advancements in patient safety protocols, technologies, and best practices. This requires regular attendance at professional development workshops, participation in continuing education programs, and proactive engagement with the latest research. Encouraging a culture of continuous improvement fosters a commitment to patient safety throughout the organization. Regular feedback and performance appraisals focused on safety practices ensure accountability and contribute to maintaining the highest standards of patient care. A system of learning from mistakes, analyzing near-misses, and implementing corrective actions is invaluable in continuously improving safety measures.

4.3 Adverse Effects Management

Managing adverse effects is crucial for ensuring patient safety and treatment success. It requires a proactive approach, starting with thorough patient assessment and a detailed understanding of the medications and therapies involved. A comprehensive medication history, including over-the-counter drugs and supplements, is essential. This allows clinicians to anticipate potential interactions and tailor treatment accordingly. This holistic approach ensures the best possible outcomes and improves adherence.

Early detection of adverse effects is paramount. Regular monitoring of vital signs, close observation for any unusual symptoms, and open communication with the patient are vital strategies. Patients should be educated to recognize and report any changes in their physical or mental state promptly. The use of standardized assessment tools can facilitate consistent and accurate tracking of potential problems. This proactive approach mitigates risks.

Once an adverse effect is identified, a systematic approach to management is critical. This involves first confirming the causal relationship between the medication or therapy and the observed effect. This requires careful review of the patient's history, medication profile, and other contributing factors. Discontinuing the offending agent is often the first step, though this decision depends on the severity of the adverse effect and the importance of the treatment itself. In some cases, dose reduction might be considered.

Symptom management is a key component. This may involve supportive care, such as pain relief medication, anti-nausea drugs, or other therapies to alleviate specific symptoms. For example, if a patient experiences muscle weakness from a medication, physiotherapy might be introduced to mitigate this issue and maintain functionality. Furthermore, appropriate referral to specialists, such as a cardiologist or dermatologist, might be needed depending on the nature of the adverse effect.

Documentation is crucial for maintaining accurate records of adverse effects, their management, and the patient's response. This ensures continuity of care and aids in future treatment decisions. Comprehensive documentation enables clinicians to track trends and patterns in adverse effects, improving their ability to predict and manage them more effectively. Furthermore, thorough documentation is essential for regulatory compliance and research purposes.

The importance of patient education cannot be overstated. Patients need to understand the potential adverse effects of their medications and therapies, as well as the signs and symptoms to watch for. Empowering patients with this knowledge encourages them to participate actively in their treatment and seek help promptly if needed. This shared responsibility fosters a strong therapeutic alliance and improves overall outcomes.

Involving family members and caregivers in the management process is equally important, especially when dealing with patients who have cognitive impairments or difficulties communicating their symptoms. They can play a vital role in monitoring the patient's condition and providing valuable insights into their experience. This collaborative approach ensures comprehensive care and supports the patient's overall well-being.

Regular review of the treatment plan is necessary to assess the effectiveness of the interventions implemented to manage the adverse effects. This review should include an evaluation of the patient's symptoms, their response to treatment, and any potential interactions between medications or therapies. Adjustments to the treatment plan may be needed, reflecting an adaptive and responsive approach to patient care. This flexibility is crucial.

Reporting of adverse effects to relevant authorities and organizations is essential for patient safety and improving healthcare systems. This practice allows for the identification of safety signals and prompt actions to prevent similar occurrences in the future. Regulatory bodies use this information to reassess the risks and benefits of medications and therapies, potentially leading to changes in prescribing practices or product labels. Reporting helps protect others.

Finally, ongoing research and monitoring are critical to better understand the causes, mechanisms, and management of adverse effects. This involves developing new diagnostic tools, exploring innovative treatment strategies, and improving our ability to predict which patients are at higher risk. By actively engaging in research and continually updating our knowledge, clinicians can better safeguard patient safety and improve healthcare overall. The pursuit of knowledge is ongoing.

4.4 Data Analysis & Interpretation

Analyzing data effectively is crucial for evaluating the success of holistic rehabilitation treatments and ensuring their safety. We need to move beyond simple observation and delve into robust statistical methods to truly understand the impact of our interventions. This involves collecting comprehensive data, meticulously documenting patient progress, and employing appropriate analytical techniques. Remember, the goal is not just to gather numbers, but to extract meaningful insights that improve patient care. Thorough documentation, including baseline assessments, regular progress notes, and outcome measures, is fundamental to this process.

Effective data collection hinges on clearly defined outcome measures. These shouldn't be generic; instead, they should be tailored to the specific goals and needs of each patient. For example, if the goal is improved mobility, then quantifiable measures like walking distance, gait speed, and range of motion are crucial. For emotional well-being, validated questionnaires assessing anxiety, depression, or quality of life are appropriate tools. The chosen measures must be reliable, valid, and sensitive enough to detect meaningful changes over time. Consistent use of these measures across all patients ensures comparability and strengthens the reliability of any subsequent analysis. The data collected must also be well-organized to avoid inconsistencies and ensure a smoother data analysis process.

Once data is collected, selecting the appropriate statistical methods is vital. The choice depends on the type of data and the research questions. For example, if comparing the effectiveness of two different treatment approaches, a t-test or ANOVA might be appropriate for continuous data. If looking at the relationship between two variables, correlation analysis is useful. For categorical data (e.g., treatment response as improved, unchanged, or worsened), chi-square tests might be suitable. However, remember that statistical significance does not necessarily imply clinical significance. A statistically significant result might represent a small, clinically unimportant difference. Therefore, interpreting the results requires clinical judgment and consideration of effect sizes, alongside the p-values.

Data interpretation isn't just about crunching numbers; it's about telling a story. We need to present our findings clearly and concisely, using tables, graphs, and concise summaries. Visual representations of data can make complex information more accessible and impactful. Bar charts, line graphs, and scatter plots can effectively illustrate trends and relationships. This is particularly helpful when reporting to other healthcare professionals, researchers, or regulatory bodies. Moreover, a clear explanation of the limitations of your study and its potential impact on generalizability needs to be included in the final report.

Furthermore, it's important to consider potential biases in the data. Selection bias can occur if participants aren't randomly assigned to treatment groups, leading to skewed results. Recall bias, where patients may inaccurately remember past events, is also a risk, especially when relying on self-reported data. Careful study design, blinding procedures, and rigorous data collection protocols can help mitigate these biases. Transparency in the reporting of these potential biases helps researchers and readers to properly interpret findings. Addressing these issues will lead to more reliable and trustworthy results in the final study.

Finally, remember that data analysis is an iterative process. Initial analyses might raise new questions or suggest further investigation. We need to be prepared to refine our methods, collect additional data if necessary, and re-evaluate our conclusions as needed. This iterative approach ensures that our findings are as robust and meaningful as possible. The end goal is to use the data to inform best practices, improve treatment protocols, and ultimately enhance patient care. Successful data analysis empowers clinicians to make evidence-based decisions and contributes to advancing the field of holistic rehabilitation. By embracing data-driven decision making, we can move closer to achieving better outcomes for all our patients, promoting a more personalized and responsive approach to treatment. This will provide the best evidence-based approach to care.

4.5 Future Directions in Research

The field of holistic rehabilitation, while showing immense promise, requires further investigation to solidify its place in mainstream healthcare. One crucial area needing exploration is the development of standardized assessment tools specifically designed for holistic interventions. Current methods often lack the sensitivity to capture the multifaceted nature of improvements observed in patients undergoing holistic therapies, making it difficult to demonstrate efficacy convincingly compared to conventional treatments. Robust, validated tools are essential for demonstrating the value of these approaches to funding bodies, policymakers, and even patients themselves, leading to greater acceptance and integration into established healthcare systems. This will require collaborative efforts between researchers, clinicians, and statisticians to ensure the instruments capture both quantitative and qualitative data, reflecting the holistic nature of the interventions.

A significant challenge lies in disentangling the effects of various components within holistic treatment plans. Often, multiple interventions are used concurrently – physiotherapy, nutritional guidance, mindfulness practices – making it hard to isolate the contribution of each element. Future research should focus on designing rigorous randomized controlled trials with carefully controlled intervention arms to determine the effectiveness of individual components and their potential synergistic interactions. This nuanced understanding will allow for the tailoring of interventions to the specific needs of individual patients, maximizing efficiency and minimizing unnecessary treatment. This approach requires a shift from broad-brush approaches to more precisely targeted therapies.

The long-term sustainability of holistic approaches also demands investigation. While immediate benefits are often observed, the long-term effects, both positive and negative, need comprehensive study. We need to understand if the improvements achieved are maintained over time, identifying potential factors contributing to sustained recovery or relapse. Longitudinal studies tracking patients over extended periods, incorporating both objective and subjective measures, are crucial to address this gap. This sustained follow-up will provide invaluable insights into the true impact of these interventions, clarifying their true role in long-term patient management.

Furthermore, the cost-effectiveness of holistic therapies compared to conventional methods requires thorough examination. While anecdotal evidence suggests potential cost savings through reduced medication use and shorter rehabilitation periods, robust economic evaluations are needed to provide strong evidence supporting its financial viability. Such analyses should consider the full spectrum of costs, encompassing direct healthcare expenditure, indirect costs like lost productivity, and the long-term societal benefits of improved patient outcomes. Only with such data can healthcare systems make informed decisions about resource allocation. This will allow for the optimization of healthcare spending, thereby improving value for money.

Equitable access to holistic therapies remains a major concern. Geographic location, socioeconomic status, and other factors create significant disparities in access to these often expensive and specialized treatments. Research should focus on developing strategies to ensure equitable distribution of holistic services. This might involve exploring telehealth options, creating community-based programs, and implementing policies to promote affordability and access for all patient populations, regardless of their background. We must actively address these inequalities to realize the full potential of these therapies, ensuring that all members of society can benefit.

Another area of needed focus involves integrating holistic and conventional approaches. Currently, there is often a dichotomy between conventional and holistic medicine, hindering their full integration in patient care. Future research should investigate the potential synergy between these approaches, exploring optimal methods for integrating different therapeutic modalities. This could involve developing collaborative care models that seamlessly combine evidence-based conventional treatments with appropriate holistic interventions. This collaborative approach will create more comprehensive and effective treatment plans. This integration promises to move beyond a simple choice between approaches and instead use the strengths of each to achieve superior patient outcomes.

Finally, we must acknowledge the significant role of patient experience and preferences. Future research should incorporate patient-centered methodologies to deeply understand the perspectives and needs of individuals undergoing holistic rehabilitation. Qualitative research, including focus groups and interviews, can provide valuable insights into how holistic therapies impact patients' lives, offering crucial data often absent from quantitative studies. Incorporating patient feedback into treatment protocols will enable us to enhance the therapeutic experience and optimize adherence, leading to better outcomes. Understanding the lived experience, therefore, is critical in developing truly holistic care.

5 Holistic Therapies: A Deep Dive

Physiotherapy, a cornerstone of holistic rehabilitation, goes beyond addressing immediate pain. It's about restoring movement, improving function, and ultimately enhancing a patient's quality of life. Consider a stroke patient struggling with impaired mobility; physiotherapy helps regain lost strength, coordination, and independence, potentially reducing their reliance on assistive devices and improving their participation in daily activities. This process involves a thorough assessment of the patient's condition, setting realistic goals, and tailoring a program of exercises and therapies to meet their specific needs. This might encompass range-of-motion exercises, strengthening activities, gait training, and the use of specialized equipment, all while constantly monitoring progress and adapting the treatment plan as needed. The impact extends beyond the physical, positively influencing mental well-being and fostering a sense of empowerment. Occupational therapy plays a vital role in enabling patients to regain their functional independence in daily life. Unlike physiotherapy's focus on physical restoration, occupational therapy centers around adapting activities and environments to support participation. For instance, a patient recovering from a traumatic brain injury may experience difficulties with cognitive functions, such as memory and attention. Occupational therapists work collaboratively with the patient, assessing their specific challenges and developing strategies to overcome them. This might involve adapting everyday tasks, such as dressing and cooking, through assistive technology or compensatory strategies. The aim is to empower individuals to perform activities of daily living safely and effectively, ultimately promoting a sense of self-sufficiency and integration back into their communities. Furthermore, occupational therapists address the psychological and emotional aspects of recovery, recognizing that participation in meaningful activities plays a crucial role in overall rehabilitation success.

Complementary therapies, often integrated within a holistic approach, offer diverse avenues for enhancing patient well-being. Acupuncture, for example, based on traditional Chinese medicine, aims to restore balance in the body's energy flow by stimulating specific points on the skin with thin needles. Its application in rehabilitation can alleviate pain, reduce inflammation, and improve mobility, particularly in conditions like chronic back pain or osteoarthritis. Massage therapy, another complementary technique, employs manual manipulation of soft tissues to relieve muscle tension, improve circulation, and promote relaxation. It can be especially beneficial in managing stress and pain associated with injury or illness. Mindfulness-based interventions, such as meditation and yoga, help patients cultivate self-awareness, manage stress, and improve emotional regulation. The evidence supporting these therapies is growing, indicating potential benefits for physical and mental health outcomes in various rehabilitation settings. However, it's crucial to acknowledge that while complementary therapies can be valuable adjuncts, they should not replace conventional medical treatments. Careful consideration should be given to their integration within a patient's overall care plan. Their successful implementation requires careful consideration of patient preferences, potential interactions with other therapies, and the availability of qualified practitioners. Thorough research into these areas can help ensure responsible and effective use, maximizing their benefit to the patient's overall health and recovery journey.

The holistic approach isn't simply about adding complementary therapies to conventional treatments; it's about a fundamental shift in perspective. It prioritizes the interconnectedness of physical, emotional, and social well-being, recognizing that these elements influence each other profoundly. Imagine a patient with chronic pain: a purely biomedical approach may focus solely on managing pain through medication. A holistic approach, on the other hand, would consider the patient's lifestyle, stress levels, social support network, and beliefs. This integrated approach might incorporate physiotherapy to address physical limitations, occupational therapy to adapt daily activities, and mindfulness techniques to manage stress, creating a more comprehensive and potentially more effective intervention strategy. This patient-centered approach empowers individuals to take an active role in their recovery, fostering a sense of control and improving their overall prognosis.

Integrating these diverse approaches requires interprofessional collaboration. Effective communication and shared decision-making between physiotherapists, occupational therapists, complementary therapists, and other healthcare professionals are paramount. This team approach allows for a comprehensive assessment of the patient's needs and the development of a personalized treatment plan that addresses all aspects of their well-being. Open communication ensures consistency in the patient's care, minimizing confusion and maximizing the synergistic effects of different therapies. Effective teamwork and coordinated effort are key to creating a seamless and supportive environment that fosters patient recovery and empowers individuals to regain their independence and quality of life. It is about creating a care approach that is not only effective but also deeply respectful of the individual's needs and preferences, acknowledging the rich tapestry of their life experiences that inevitably contribute to their path to recovery. Only through such a comprehensive and collaborative approach can we truly leverage the immense potential of holistic therapies for better patient outcomes.

5.1 Physiotherapy & its Applications

Physiotherapy, a cornerstone of holistic rehabilitation, uses movement and exercise to restore function, alleviate pain, and improve overall well-being. Its applications are incredibly diverse, spanning a wide spectrum of conditions and patient populations. From the acute injury sustained on the sports field to the chronic pain associated with aging, physiotherapy provides targeted interventions aimed at restoring mobility, strength, and flexibility. We'll explore how this multifaceted therapy addresses various needs.

The initial assessment is crucial. A thorough evaluation involves a detailed medical history, a physical examination focusing on range of motion, muscle strength, and any pain or limitations, and often includes imaging studies like X-rays or MRIs to clarify the diagnosis. This comprehensive approach provides a personalized treatment plan, tailoring exercises and modalities to the individual's specific needs and capabilities. It's not a one-size-fits-all approach; rather, it's adaptable and responsive to the patient's progress.

Manual therapy, a key element of physiotherapy, involves hands-on techniques to address musculoskeletal issues. Soft tissue mobilization, joint manipulation, and trigger point therapy are just some examples. These manual techniques aim to improve joint mobility, reduce muscle tension, and alleviate pain directly at the source. Combined with therapeutic exercises, this approach provides a powerful synergy, promoting both immediate pain relief and long-term functional improvements. The therapist's expertise in assessing the patient's specific needs and selecting the most appropriate manual techniques is vital for success.

Therapeutic exercise, designed to improve strength, flexibility, and endurance, forms the backbone of most physiotherapy programs. Exercises are carefully selected based on the patient's condition and goals, gradually increasing in intensity and complexity as they progress. This progressive approach minimizes the risk of re-injury and maximizes the potential for functional gains. There are exercises for every level of ability. Home exercise programs are also critical, reinforcing the gains made during therapy sessions and fostering patient independence. This self-management aspect empowers patients to take an active role in their recovery.

Beyond the exercise and manual techniques, physiotherapy incorporates other modalities like electrotherapy, ultrasound, and heat or cold therapy. Electrotherapy uses electrical currents to stimulate muscles, reduce pain, and promote healing. Ultrasound uses high-frequency sound waves to promote tissue healing and reduce inflammation. Heat and cold therapies, applied strategically, can manage pain and inflammation. The choice of modality depends on the specific condition and the patient's response. The correct application of these modalities demands a high level of expertise.

The scope of physiotherapy extends beyond individual treatments. A crucial aspect involves patient education and self-management strategies. Physios teach patients about their condition, proper body mechanics, and strategies for preventing future injuries. This educational component empowers patients to make informed decisions about their healthcare and to take active responsibility for their recovery. The goal is not just to treat the current problem but also to equip the individual with the knowledge and tools for long-term health and wellness.

Physiotherapy's applications are broad, encompassing various age groups and conditions. In pediatric physiotherapy, interventions focus on developmental milestones, addressing conditions like cerebral palsy or musculoskeletal deformities. Geriatric physiotherapy addresses age-related changes, focusing on improving balance, mobility, and preventing falls. In sports medicine, physiotherapy plays a critical role in rehabilitation from injuries, optimizing athletic performance and preventing future re-injuries. And in neurological rehabilitation, it helps patients recover from strokes, spinal cord injuries, or other neurological conditions, focusing on restoring motor function and independence.

The ethical considerations are paramount. Informed consent is central; patients must understand the nature of the treatment, its benefits and risks, and the alternatives available. Confidentiality and respect for patient autonomy are also critical components. The therapist must maintain the highest ethical standards, ensuring transparency, honesty, and respect for the patient's beliefs and values. The patient-therapist relationship is grounded in trust, mutual respect, and shared decision-making.

Finally, the effectiveness of physiotherapy is supported by robust research. Studies consistently demonstrate its efficacy in treating a wide range of conditions, showing improvements in functional outcomes, pain reduction, and quality of life. Integrating physiotherapy into a holistic rehabilitation plan provides a comprehensive, patient-centered approach that optimizes recovery and enhances overall well-being. The benefits extend beyond the immediate treatment period, fostering long-term health and independence. The future of physiotherapy involves ongoing research, technological advancements, and an increasing integration with other holistic therapies.

5.2 Occupational Therapy's Role

Occupational therapy plays a vital role in holistic rehabilitation, focusing on enabling individuals to participate in meaningful activities of daily living. It's not simply about regaining physical function; it's about restoring independence and improving overall quality of life. This involves a thorough assessment of a patient's strengths, weaknesses, and goals, leading to personalized intervention plans. These plans address a wide range of challenges, from fine motor skill deficits to cognitive impairments, adapting tasks and environments to promote successful engagement.

A core aspect of occupational therapy is its emphasis on adaptive techniques and assistive technology. This means finding creative ways to modify tasks or using specialized tools to help individuals perform activities that might otherwise be difficult or impossible. For instance, a person with arthritis might benefit from adapted kitchen utensils, while someone with limited mobility could use a specialized dressing aid. The goal isn't to simply complete the task, but to do it efficiently and with a sense of accomplishment, boosting self-esteem and independence.

The therapeutic process itself isn't confined to one-on-one sessions. Occupational therapists frequently work collaboratively with patients' families and caregivers, providing education and support to ensure that interventions can continue effectively outside of the clinical setting. This holistic approach recognizes the profound impact of social and environmental factors on recovery, extending the therapeutic reach beyond the treatment room. Such collaborations foster a shared understanding of the patient's needs and goals, leading to more effective and sustainable outcomes.

Ethical considerations are central to occupational therapy practice. Respect for patient autonomy is paramount; treatment plans are always developed in close consultation with individuals, ensuring they are actively involved in shaping their own recovery journey. Confidentiality is strictly maintained, protecting sensitive information and fostering trust between therapist and patient. Furthermore, occupational therapists strive to provide equitable access to care, regardless of a patient's socioeconomic background or other demographics, acknowledging that everyone deserves the opportunity to reach their full potential.

The assessment process within occupational therapy is far-reaching and multifaceted. It extends beyond simple observation of motor skills; therapists carefully consider a patient's cognitive abilities, emotional state, and social context. The tools employed can range from standardized tests measuring specific functions to informal observations of daily activities, tailoring the assessment to the individual's specific needs and situation. This comprehensive approach offers a nuanced understanding of the patient's challenges, informing the development of highly targeted and effective interventions. Data collection methods might include observations, interviews, and the use of standardized questionnaires, providing a rich source of information to inform treatment planning and track progress.

Occupational therapy's impact extends far beyond the physical restoration of function. It addresses the psychological and emotional aspects of recovery, recognizing the significant impact that illness or injury can have on a person's sense of self-worth and identity. Therapists often incorporate activities that promote self-esteem and emotional regulation, helping patients to cope with the challenges of rehabilitation and rebuild their lives. This aspect is crucial, as the restoration of emotional well-being is inextricably linked to the overall success of the rehabilitation process. Support groups, stress management techniques, and cognitive behavioral therapy may be incorporated depending on the patient's needs and goals, highlighting the comprehensive nature of occupational therapy's approach.

Measuring the effectiveness of occupational therapy requires a multi-pronged approach. Quantitative measures, such as the improvement in range of motion or the ability to perform specific tasks, provide objective data. However, these must be complemented by qualitative assessments that capture the subjective experience of the patient. This is crucial because a person's perception of their progress and level of satisfaction is a key indicator of successful rehabilitation. The effectiveness and value are not only measured in objective improvements but also in how the intervention helps them engage in meaningful life activities. The role of occupational therapy is constantly evolving, incorporating new technologies and treatment approaches. Virtual reality, for instance, offers innovative opportunities for practicing functional tasks in a safe and controlled environment. Similarly, advancements in assistive technology continually expand the possibilities for enhancing independence and participation. Ongoing professional development is crucial for occupational therapists to remain at the forefront of these advancements and provide the best possible care to their patients. Adaptability and a commitment to lifelong learning are essential for ensuring that occupational therapy remains a highly effective and relevant component of holistic rehabilitation. The field is constantly shaped by rigorous research and evidence-based practices, leading to the integration of innovative and highly effective treatment methods.

5.3 Complementary Therapies

Acupuncture, a cornerstone of Traditional Chinese Medicine, involves inserting thin needles into specific points on the body. The purported mechanism involves stimulating energy flow (Qi) and reducing pain by releasing endorphins. While its efficacy for certain musculoskeletal conditions has shown some promising results in randomized controlled trials, more research is needed to establish clear guidelines for its application across diverse patient populations. The ethical considerations revolve around ensuring practitioner competence and transparency about the limitations of evidence regarding its effectiveness. Clinicians should always prioritize evidence-based practices while maintaining open communication with patients about both the potential benefits and risks. Furthermore, cultural sensitivity is paramount, as acupuncture's cultural roots can influence patient expectations and perceptions of its efficacy.

Massage therapy, a widely used complementary therapy, utilizes various techniques to manipulate soft tissues, promoting relaxation, reducing muscle tension, and improving circulation. Its benefits have been demonstrated in reducing pain and improving range of motion in patients with musculoskeletal disorders. However, the effectiveness can vary depending on the therapist's skill, the type of massage, and the individual patient's response. Safety concerns are generally minimal when performed by a qualified practitioner, but potential risks like bruising or aggravation of underlying conditions must be carefully considered and addressed. Ethical practice includes obtaining informed consent, explaining the procedure and potential side effects, and respecting patient boundaries. Proper training and licensing for massage therapists are crucial to ensure the safety and efficacy of the therapy.

Mindfulness-based interventions, including meditation and yoga, are increasingly incorporated into rehabilitation programs. These practices aim to cultivate present moment awareness, reducing stress and improving emotional regulation. Studies have shown their effectiveness in managing chronic pain, improving sleep quality, and reducing anxiety and depression – common challenges faced by individuals undergoing rehabilitation. However, the mechanisms through which these benefits are achieved are not fully understood, highlighting the need for further research. Ethical considerations focus on ensuring patients are comfortable with the mindfulness techniques employed, respecting their religious or spiritual beliefs, and tailoring interventions to their individual needs and preferences. Care must be taken to avoid implying that mindfulness can replace established medical treatments. The practitioner's role is to guide and support the patient, empowering them to develop skills for self-management, rather than acting as a healer in the traditional sense.

Yoga, a practice that combines physical postures, breathing techniques, and meditation, offers a holistic approach to health and well-being. Its use in rehabilitation shows promise in improving flexibility, strength, balance, and overall functional capacity in patients recovering from various conditions. For example, studies show its beneficial effects in managing chronic pain conditions like fibromyalgia. However, it's crucial to adapt the practice to individual capabilities and limitations, carefully modifying poses to avoid injury. Ethical concerns center around proper training of instructors, clear communication about potential risks, and considering patient's physical limitations and any contraindications. Informed consent is crucial, ensuring the patient understands what to expect and has the option to opt out at any time. Moreover, ensuring accessibility for people with various physical abilities is a key ethical consideration. Modifications and adaptations of poses are necessary to ensure inclusivity and maximize safety.

The integration of these complementary therapies into rehabilitation must adhere to rigorous ethical and clinical standards. Effective integration requires collaboration between healthcare professionals, ensuring appropriate referrals, communication, and shared decision-making. The use of complementary therapies should never replace conventional medical treatment without thorough assessment and consideration of the individual's health status. Instead, a thoughtful approach involves combining conventional medicine with appropriate complementary therapies to enhance patient outcomes. It's about providing comprehensive care that respects individual needs and preferences while maintaining the highest standards of clinical practice and ethical conduct.

6 Patient Recovery and its Measurement

Measuring a patient's recovery isn't simply about charting physical progress; it's about understanding the holistic journey back to well-being. We need to move beyond solely quantifiable metrics and embrace a broader perspective, incorporating qualitative data and understanding the nuances of each individual's experience. A fractured tibia heals according to a predictable timeline, but the emotional impact of that injury, the anxiety surrounding mobility limitations, and the subsequent adjustment to daily life – these are factors equally deserving of careful consideration.

Functional outcome measures are crucial, providing objective data on improvements in strength, range of motion, and activities of daily living. The 6-minute walk test, for instance, objectively measures cardiovascular fitness, while assessments of grip strength quantify upper body functionality. These tests offer concrete evidence of progress, informing clinicians and allowing for objective tracking of the recovery journey. However, relying solely on these numbers ignores the rich tapestry of a person's lived experience.

Consider, for example, a patient recovering from a stroke. Functional outcome measures might track improvements in arm movement or speech articulation.

Yet, these numbers don't fully capture the frustration of battling aphasia, the emotional toll of lost independence, or the resilience demonstrated in daily struggle. To fully understand the recovery process, we must engage with the patient's narrative. Gathering qualitative data, whether through structured interviews or open-ended questionnaires, allows clinicians to understand how the patient perceives their recovery. It gives voice to their experiences, frustrations, and triumphs.

This qualitative data provides invaluable insight. We can learn about the psychological and emotional barriers to recovery that aren't captured in simple measurements. For instance, a patient might demonstrate significant improvements in physical function but still struggle with anxiety or depression, hindering their overall progress. Understanding these emotional challenges allows clinicians to tailor interventions to address both the physical and mental aspects of recovery. This holistic approach, intertwining objective metrics with subjective experiences, leads to more effective and compassionate care.

Gathering meaningful qualitative data requires careful planning. Questions should be open-ended, avoiding leading prompts that could bias responses. The interviewer's approach should be empathetic, creating a safe space for the patient to share their thoughts and feelings openly. Moreover, the timing of these interviews should be carefully considered; some patients may find it more helpful to reflect on their recovery at different stages. It is essential to respect the patient's autonomy and to ensure their comfort throughout the interview process.

The integration of quantitative and qualitative data isn't just about adding extra layers of information; it's about crafting a more complete understanding of the patient's journey. By analyzing both the numbers and the narrative, we can identify patterns, highlight areas where additional support may be needed, and refine interventions to better serve patients. This comprehensive approach leads to a more personalized and effective recovery process, fostering a greater sense of collaboration and empowerment for those navigating the challenges of rehabilitation.

Furthermore, the use of technology has dramatically changed the landscape of data collection in rehabilitation settings. Wearable sensors, for instance, can continuously monitor various aspects of a patient's activity, providing detailed and objective data on their movements and physical exertion. This continuous monitoring, combined with regular qualitative feedback, offers a particularly rich dataset that can inform treatment decisions and track progress with precision.

Analyzing this combined data requires advanced statistical techniques and a keen understanding of both quantitative and qualitative research methods. The synthesis of these various data points provides a much richer and holistic representation of the recovery process than either type of data alone can achieve. This comprehensive understanding isn't simply about improving patient outcomes; it is about demonstrating respect for the complex and multifaceted nature of the human experience of recovery.

Finally, the analysis and interpretation of patient data should not be confined to the immediate clinical team. The findings should be shared across wider professional networks, enriching the broader understanding of recovery processes and informing future research. By openly sharing data and insights, we contribute to a collective knowledge base, constantly refining our approaches to patient care and promoting the best possible recovery outcomes. This ongoing collaborative effort is crucial to the ongoing evolution of rehabilitation practices. This commitment to transparency and collaboration is vital for continuous improvement within the field. The ultimate goal is not just to measure recovery, but to enhance it, understanding that the human experience is far richer and more complex than any single data point can capture.

6.1 Assessing Functional Outcomes

The cornerstone of successful rehabilitation lies in accurately assessing functional outcomes. This isn't simply about measuring strength or range of motion; it's about understanding the patient's ability to perform everyday tasks and participate in life's activities. We need to move beyond quantifiable data and delve into the patient's lived experience, acknowledging that recovery is a deeply personal journey.

A comprehensive assessment involves a multi-faceted approach. Standardized assessments, like the Barthel Index or the Functional Independence Measure (FIM), provide objective data on activities of daily living (ADLs). These tools offer a quantifiable metric of improvement, crucial for tracking progress and demonstrating the efficacy of interventions. However, relying solely on these metrics would present an incomplete picture.

Consider, for instance, a patient recovering from a stroke. While the FIM may show improvement in their ability to dress themselves, it may not capture their frustration with the time it takes or the decreased dexterity impacting their ability to button their shirt. Their experience, their feelings of independence, self-efficacy, and confidence are vital to understanding their true functional outcome. This requires incorporating qualitative measures.

Qualitative data gathering methods, such as semi-structured interviews or focus groups, provide valuable insights into the patient's perspective. Open-ended questions allow patients to express their experiences, challenges, and aspirations in their own words, revealing nuances that standardized assessments might miss.

For example, a patient might describe regaining independence in their mobility but still struggling with the emotional impact of their injury.

Integrating both quantitative and qualitative methods creates a rich and nuanced understanding of functional outcomes. Triangulation—comparing data from multiple sources—enhances the reliability and validity of the assessment. Analyzing both FIM scores and patient narratives can reveal discrepancies and unexpected insights, refining our understanding of the patient's recovery journey. These techniques allow clinicians to tailor their treatment plans to effectively address both the physical and emotional aspects of rehabilitation.

Furthermore, the assessment process must consider the context of the patient's life. Their social environment, cultural background, and personal goals significantly influence their recovery trajectory. A patient's home environment, for example, may present challenges that impact their functional independence. Similarly, cultural beliefs about health and recovery might shape a patient's expectations and engagement with rehabilitation. Therefore, a comprehensive assessment must account for these diverse contexts.

The inclusion of caregivers and family members in the assessment process is also crucial. Their perspectives provide valuable information about the patient's pre-morbid functioning and current limitations. They can provide detailed accounts of the patient's progress at home, highlighting challenges that might not be evident in a clinical setting. This collaborative approach ensures that the assessment is comprehensive and accounts for all relevant factors influencing the patient's recovery.

The ultimate goal is not simply to measure functional improvements but to guide the development of personalized rehabilitation programs. By combining objective data with qualitative insights and considering the patient's unique context, clinicians can create effective and patient-centered interventions that promote both physical and emotional well-being. This holistic approach ensures that the patient's journey towards recovery is as meaningful and successful as possible. We aim not just for measurable improvements, but for a restoration of meaningful engagement with life—a truly holistic perspective on rehabilitation. The impact goes beyond physical recovery to encompass emotional, psychological, and social wellbeing. This process also necessitates regular reassessment to capture fluctuations in functional status and adapt interventions accordingly. A dynamic approach is essential, recognizing that rehabilitation is not a linear process but rather a journey involving highs and lows.

6.2 Qualitative Patient Feedback

Qualitative patient feedback offers invaluable insights beyond numerical data. It allows us to understand the lived experience of recovery, capturing the nuances of a patient's journey that quantitative measures often miss. This richer, more textured understanding is crucial for tailoring treatment plans to individual needs, ultimately leading to improved outcomes and patient satisfaction. Think about the subtle shifts in mood, the unexpected challenges, the moments of breakthrough—these are rarely captured by a simple functional assessment. Instead, open-ended questions and focused interviews allow us to access this crucial information, enriching our overall comprehension of the rehabilitation process.

The process of gathering qualitative data requires careful planning and execution. We need to choose appropriate methods, such as semi-structured interviews, focus groups, or even open-ended questionnaires, selecting the technique most suitable for the specific aims and the patient population. Regardless of the chosen method, it's paramount to create a safe and trusting environment, ensuring patients feel comfortable sharing their experiences honestly and without fear of judgment. A skilled interviewer should use active listening techniques, and create an atmosphere of genuine respect and understanding. Sensitive topics might arise during those conversations; therefore, it is critical to approach them with appropriate empathy and professional boundaries.

Analyzing qualitative data differs significantly from the more straightforward processes involved in interpreting quantitative results. Instead of relying on statistical analysis, this requires a more nuanced and interpretive approach. Thematic analysis, grounded theory, and narrative analysis are among the methods used to identify patterns and recurring themes within the data collected. This iterative process involves careful reading and rereading of transcripts, identifying recurring patterns, and then categorizing and interpreting those themes. It is essential to note that this process is subjective. Therefore, using a robust framework, having clear criteria, and involving multiple researchers can assist in mitigating any biases. The aim here is to synthesize the data and provide a rich, descriptive account that captures the essence of the patient experience.

The ethical considerations associated with qualitative data collection are also important. Informed consent is paramount—patients must understand the purpose of the study, how their data will be used, and their right to withdraw at any time. Confidentiality and anonymity are also critical, ensuring that patient identities are protected throughout the research process. Data must be stored securely and accessed only by authorized personnel. The use of pseudonyms and the careful redaction of identifying information are vital steps to guarantee the patient's right to privacy. Researchers must adhere to strict ethical guidelines throughout the research process, and it is essential that any findings are reported responsibly, providing a balanced perspective that acknowledges both positive and negative aspects.

Using qualitative patient feedback effectively involves translating the findings into actionable steps for improving care. The identified themes and patterns can inform the development of new treatment protocols, identify areas for improvement in communication or patient support, or even lead to changes in the overall approach to rehabilitation. For example, recurrent themes might highlight the inadequacy of emotional support or the need for more tailored approaches to physical therapy. Sharing these findings, not just within the clinical team, but also with patients themselves, and with colleagues, demonstrates a commitment to transparency and continuous improvement. It helps foster a culture of feedback that prioritizes the patient's experience and promotes the ongoing development of patient-centered care. A detailed report, which should include a summary of the methodology, the identified themes, as well as any recommendations for practice changes, is vital for this stage. It allows for a deeper analysis of strengths and weaknesses, ensuring the highest quality of care possible.

Beyond its direct application to individual patient care, qualitative feedback contributes significantly to the broader field of rehabilitation research. By providing rich contextual information, it allows researchers to explore the complex interplay of factors that influence recovery, leading to a more nuanced and complete understanding of the patient journey. This knowledge, in turn, can inform the development of more effective and patient-centered rehabilitation programs and can generate hypotheses for future quantitative research. Moreover, this can lead to greater efficiency within the system. By refining and improving existing protocols, we can increase the effectiveness of treatment, ensuring the most optimal recovery for every patient and ultimately enhancing the overall outcome of the rehabilitation process. Publishing these findings in professional journals promotes the sharing of best practice across the rehabilitation community.

7 Conclusion and Future Perspectives

The integration of holistic and conventional care represents a paradigm shift in rehabilitation, promising enhanced patient outcomes and improved quality of life. This synergistic approach acknowledges the interconnectedness of physical, emotional, and social well-being, moving beyond a solely biomedical model to a more comprehensive understanding of recovery. Successful implementation hinges on overcoming challenges such as interprofessional collaboration, standardized assessment tools for holistic interventions, and clear reimbursement guidelines. However, the rewards are substantial; imagine a future where patients experience faster recovery times, reduced reliance on pharmaceuticals, and greater personal agency in their healing journey.

Addressing the persistent disparities in access to quality rehabilitation, regardless of socioeconomic status, geographic location, or cultural background, is paramount. We must actively work towards dismantling systemic barriers that prevent equitable access. This requires policy changes, innovative funding models, and community-based programs that bridge geographical and socioeconomic divides. Furthermore, culturally sensitive rehabilitation practices must be developed and implemented, ensuring that treatment plans are tailored to individual needs and beliefs. The path forward demands proactive engagement from healthcare systems, policymakers, and communities alike.

Ethical considerations remain central to holistic rehabilitation. While respecting patient autonomy and informed consent are cornerstones of ethical practice, the integration of complementary therapies necessitates careful evaluation of their safety and efficacy. Transparency, clear communication with patients about both benefits and risks, and thorough documentation are essential to maintain ethical standards. Moreover, robust mechanisms for reporting and addressing adverse events are crucial, ensuring patient safety remains paramount. Continued dialogue and collaboration among healthcare professionals, ethicists, and patient advocacy groups will be vital in shaping ethical guidelines for this evolving field.

Future research needs to prioritize the rigorous evaluation of holistic therapies within randomized controlled trials, establishing clear evidence of efficacy for various conditions and demographics. Further research is needed to investigate the long-term effects of integrating holistic and conventional approaches, and to understand the cost-effectiveness of such integrated care models. Exploring the mechanisms through which holistic therapies exert their effects will enhance our understanding of their therapeutic value and may lead to the development of even more effective rehabilitation strategies. This requires a collaborative effort between researchers, clinicians, and patients.

The journey towards a more holistic and equitable rehabilitation system is an ongoing process. It necessitates a collective commitment to continuous learning, adaptive practices, and ongoing evaluation. By embracing innovation, prioritizing ethical principles, and valuing patient-centered care, we can create a future where rehabilitation services are accessible, effective, and tailored to meet the unique needs of each individual, fostering true recovery and enhanced well-being across all demographics. The potential for transformation is immense, offering hope for improved lives and healthier communities. The future of rehabilitation lies in the collaborative pursuit of excellence, driven by a profound commitment to patient-centered care and ethical practice. This involves ongoing research, dedicated education, and steadfast advocacy. Let us work together to build a brighter future for rehabilitation.

7.1 Integrating Holistic and Conventional Care

Successful integration of holistic and conventional care requires a nuanced understanding of both approaches and a commitment to patient-centered care. It's not about choosing one over the other, but rather weaving them together to create a synergistic treatment plan. For example, a patient recovering from a stroke might benefit from conventional physiotherapy to regain motor skills while simultaneously incorporating mindfulness techniques to manage stress and anxiety, common obstacles to recovery. This integrated approach acknowledges the interconnectedness of physical, mental, and emotional well-being.

The key lies in open communication and collaboration between healthcare professionals. Physicians, physiotherapists, occupational therapists, and complementary therapy practitioners must work together, sharing information and coordinating treatment plans. Regular team meetings, where each member contributes their unique perspective, are crucial. This ensures the patient receives a comprehensive and coordinated approach, avoiding duplication and potential conflicts between treatments. The shared understanding prevents contradictory advice and fosters a supportive, collaborative atmosphere.

Effective integration demands meticulous record-keeping. Detailed documentation of both conventional and holistic treatments, patient responses, and any adverse effects is paramount. This comprehensive record allows for a clear picture of the patient's progress and facilitates informed decision-making. Moreover, robust documentation protects both the patient and the practitioners from potential legal issues, providing a transparent and accountable approach to care. This detailed information serves as a vital foundation for future research and improvements within the field.

Patient autonomy is central to this integrative model. Patients should actively participate in shaping their treatment plan, understanding the rationale behind each intervention, and having the opportunity to express their preferences and concerns. Shared decision-making ensures the treatment aligns with the patient's values and goals, leading to greater adherence and improved outcomes. Empowering patients in this way enhances their sense of control over their recovery journey and contributes positively to their overall well-being.

Implementing this model requires addressing potential challenges. One significant hurdle is the lack of reimbursement for some holistic therapies within conventional healthcare systems. Advocating for policy changes that recognize the value and effectiveness of integrated care is crucial. This involves demonstrating the cost-effectiveness of holistic therapies through robust research that quantifies their positive impact on patient outcomes, thus showing long-term cost savings.

Furthermore, training healthcare professionals in both conventional and holistic methods is essential. Developing interprofessional education programs can foster collaboration and shared understanding, ensuring all practitioners are equipped to contribute to this integrative approach. This approach to education ensures healthcare providers can effectively communicate with patients and other professionals involved in their care, avoiding any misunderstandings or potential conflicts.

Another significant obstacle is navigating the varying levels of evidence supporting different holistic therapies. While some therapies have strong research backing, others remain less rigorously studied. A balanced approach involves acknowledging this evidence gap and prioritizing interventions with robust evidence, whilst acknowledging the potential benefits of those with less comprehensive research available, provided there is no risk to the patient. Open and honest communication with patients regarding the evidence base is vital.

Ultimately, the successful integration of holistic and conventional care promises a more patient-centered, effective, and ethical approach to rehabilitation. By fostering collaboration, prioritizing patient autonomy, and addressing the associated challenges, healthcare systems can revolutionize patient recovery, improving both physical and mental well-being. This is essential for ensuring truly effective and equitable healthcare across all demographics. Continual research and evaluation are critical to refine and improve this integrated model, ensuring it remains at the forefront of patient care innovation. The future of rehabilitation lies in this collaborative and holistic approach.

7.2 Challenges and Opportunities

The integration of holistic and conventional approaches presents a significant challenge, demanding a paradigm shift in healthcare delivery. Successfully navigating this transition requires overcoming ingrained biases within the medical establishment, fostering interdisciplinary collaboration, and developing robust systems for data collection and analysis that encompass both qualitative and quantitative measures. This necessitates a dedicated effort to train healthcare professionals in both conventional and holistic techniques, ensuring they possess the necessary skills to provide integrated care. The cost-effectiveness of such integrated models also needs careful evaluation, comparing outcomes and resource utilization against purely conventional approaches. Financial barriers to accessing holistic therapies must be addressed, possibly through insurance coverage reform or government subsidies, to ensure equitable access. Furthermore, research into the cost-effectiveness and long-term efficacy of integrated approaches is paramount. This is crucial for securing ongoing funding and widespread adoption.

Developing standardized protocols and outcome measures for holistic therapies poses a considerable hurdle. Unlike conventional medicine, where standardized assessment tools are widely accepted, the diversity of holistic practices necessitates the creation of new, rigorous, and reliable evaluation methods. These measures must not only capture physical improvements but also incorporate the subjective experiences of patients regarding their quality of life, emotional well-being, and overall sense of recovery. Without these, the effectiveness of holistic interventions will remain difficult to objectively demonstrate. This lack of standardization can hinder the acceptance of these therapies within mainstream healthcare, despite their potential benefits. Establishing clearly defined parameters for training and certification of holistic practitioners is equally crucial, ensuring consistent quality of care and upholding professional standards.

However, the opportunities stemming from this integration are immense. Holistic rehabilitation offers the potential to significantly improve patient outcomes, reduce reliance on pharmaceuticals with their associated side effects, and enhance the overall quality of life. By addressing the whole person—physical, emotional, and spiritual—we move beyond simply treating symptoms to promoting genuine healing and well-being. This holistic approach can lead to a more patient-centered model of care, fostering a stronger therapeutic alliance and empowering individuals in their recovery journey. The integration of these approaches has the potential to radically change our understanding of rehabilitation. We can move away from a fragmented, disease-focused model to a comprehensive approach that prioritizes prevention, wellness, and sustained recovery.

The potential for improved patient adherence to treatment plans presents a compelling opportunity. Holistic therapies, which often emphasize patient empowerment and self-management, can foster greater engagement in the rehabilitation process. The participatory nature of these interventions promotes a sense of ownership, leading to increased motivation and improved adherence to prescribed regimens. Furthermore, personalized treatment plans tailored to individual needs and preferences are inherently more sustainable than generic approaches, boosting compliance and enhancing outcomes. This enhanced engagement also has implications for reducing healthcare costs, particularly in the long run, by minimizing the need for repeated interventions or hospitalizations.

The integration of technology into holistic practices presents a particularly exciting opportunity. Wearable sensors, telehealth platforms, and virtual reality applications can enhance the delivery and monitoring of various therapies, improving access and expanding the reach of these services, particularly in underserved communities. This technological integration can also facilitate data collection for research, allowing for a more thorough understanding of the efficacy and safety of holistic interventions. Furthermore, the development of sophisticated data analysis tools can help to personalize treatment plans even further, optimizing outcomes for individual patients. This move towards digitally-assisted care can also transform how we train future healthcare professionals. By integrating these technologies into educational curricula, we can prepare a new generation of healthcare providers who are adept at delivering integrated, technology-enhanced care.

Addressing the challenges and maximizing the opportunities requires a collaborative effort among healthcare professionals, researchers, policymakers, and patients themselves. Open communication, mutual respect, and a shared commitment to evidence-based practice are fundamental to successful integration. By working together, we can shape a future where holistic and conventional approaches work in synergy, creating a more effective, equitable, and patient-centered healthcare system. The collective responsibility lies in fostering an environment where innovation thrives, evidence-based practices are prioritized, and the individual well-being of every patient is paramount. This necessitates investment in research and training, alongside policy reforms that support the integration of these vital approaches.

7.3 Advancing Ethical Practices

Maintaining ethical standards is paramount in holistic rehabilitation. Our commitment to patient well-being transcends mere physical recovery; it necessitates a deep respect for individual autonomy and dignity. This means actively fostering open communication, ensuring patients fully understand their treatment options, and empowering them to make informed decisions aligned with their values and preferences. Transparency is key; patients must have access to clear, concise information about their condition, potential risks, and alternative therapies. We must champion the rights of vulnerable populations, ensuring equitable access to high-quality care irrespective of socioeconomic status, race, ethnicity, or any other demographic factor.

The principle of informed consent acts as the cornerstone of ethical practice. It's not just about obtaining a signature on a form; rather, it's about creating a collaborative relationship built on trust and mutual understanding. This involves presenting information in a readily comprehensible manner, tailoring our communication style to each patient's unique needs and literacy levels. We must actively check for comprehension, ensuring that patients feel empowered to ask questions and voice concerns without fear of judgment or reprisal. This also extends to the careful consideration and management of potential conflicts of interest and maintaining strict professional boundaries at all times.

Protecting patient confidentiality and privacy is non-negotiable. Stringent adherence to data protection regulations and ethical guidelines is essential. We must safeguard sensitive patient information, employing robust security measures to prevent unauthorized access or disclosure. This includes securing physical files, encrypting electronic records, and adhering to strict protocols for data sharing and exchange. Respect for privacy extends beyond data security; it encompasses the sensitive handling of personal information during conversations, both within the healthcare team and during interactions with family members or other parties. Maintaining discretion and only sharing information on a need-to-know basis is pivotal. Our obligation to confidentiality extends beyond the direct care setting, also encompassing our social media activity and any other public interactions where patient identifiable details might appear.

Equitable access to care requires a commitment to addressing systemic inequalities that often limit access to holistic rehabilitation services for certain demographic groups. This calls for proactive steps to identify and eliminate barriers such as affordability, geographical location, cultural disparities, and language barriers. We must advocate for policies and practices that promote equitable distribution of resources and ensure that all patients, regardless of their background, have equal opportunities to benefit from high-quality holistic care. Collaborating with community organizations, health policymakers, and diverse healthcare professionals is vital to successfully achieving these objectives. Building trust within communities we serve, through culturally sensitive approaches and language support systems, is central to breaking down potential barriers. Advancing ethical practices in holistic rehabilitation necessitates continuous professional development and a commitment to ongoing reflection. Staying abreast of evolving ethical guidelines, engaging in reflective practice, and actively seeking feedback from patients and colleagues are crucial steps. Participating in workshops, attending conferences, and pursuing further education will help practitioners update their knowledge and skills. The implementation of robust ethical review boards within holistic rehabilitation centers can help ensure compliance with established standards and prevent the potential for ethical breaches. Ultimately, embracing ethical practice is not just a matter of compliance but a profound commitment to delivering compassionate, just, and patient-centered care. It's about creating a healing environment where trust, respect, and dignity form the very foundation of our work.

7.4 Promoting Equitable Access

Geographic location significantly impacts access to quality rehabilitation services. Rural communities often lack the specialized facilities and trained professionals found in urban centers, creating disparities in care. This geographical inequality is compounded by socioeconomic factors; individuals in lower-income brackets may face financial barriers preventing them from accessing even basic rehabilitation, regardless of their proximity to healthcare providers. Insurance coverage plays a crucial role, with many individuals lacking adequate coverage or facing high out-of-pocket costs that deter them from seeking necessary rehabilitation. This creates a system where access is not equitable, but rather a privilege determined by geography, socioeconomic status, and insurance coverage. Consequently, individuals in marginalized communities experience poorer outcomes, highlighting the urgent need for policy changes and resource allocation strategies to bridge these gaps.

Transportation presents another significant hurdle, particularly for those with mobility limitations. Lack of access to reliable and affordable transportation can make attending even routine rehabilitation appointments extremely challenging, potentially leading to missed appointments and compromised treatment plans. This problem is especially prevalent in rural areas with limited public transportation options. Creative solutions, such as telehealth initiatives and mobile rehabilitation units, could help address this transportation barrier and improve access to care for those facing mobility challenges and residing in areas with limited transportation options. Such innovative solutions demonstrate how resourcefulness can combat inequitable access to care.

Cultural factors also influence access to and engagement with rehabilitation services. Language barriers can hinder effective communication between healthcare providers and patients, leading to misunderstandings and treatment delays. Cultural beliefs and practices may also affect patients' willingness to seek or engage with specific rehabilitation approaches, potentially leading to underutilization of available resources. Therefore, culturally sensitive rehabilitation programs and the use of interpreters are essential to ensuring that services are accessible and effective for diverse patient populations. Providers who lack cultural competency risk alienating those they aim to help, further entrenching inequality.

Furthermore, the availability of culturally appropriate rehabilitation services is frequently overlooked. This inadequacy of cultural competency extends beyond simple language translation. It necessitates a deep understanding and respect for the patient's beliefs, values, and practices. Incorporating traditional healing methods alongside conventional rehabilitation techniques, where appropriate, can enhance patient engagement and improve treatment outcomes. The integration of cultural sensitivity within the broader framework of equitable access is fundamental to fostering trust and promoting successful recovery. Without considering these intricate cultural nuances, any attempt at equitable access falls short.

Effective advocacy and community outreach play a vital role in promoting equitable access. Raising awareness about available services, particularly within underserved communities, is crucial for encouraging participation. Establishing partnerships with community organizations and leaders can help build trust and facilitate access to care for marginalized groups. Proactive engagement with community stakeholders ensures the dissemination of information through trusted channels and addresses the specific needs and concerns of diverse populations, fostering inclusivity within the rehabilitation process itself. Only through meaningful collaboration can genuine equitable access be achieved.

Policy changes are imperative to address systemic inequities in access. Expanding healthcare coverage to include comprehensive rehabilitation services is essential, particularly for vulnerable populations. Investing in the development of community-based rehabilitation programs in underserved areas is also crucial to increase access for individuals in remote regions or those facing transportation barriers. These policy-level interventions require not only funding but also a committed effort to challenge and change long-standing systemic disadvantages affecting rehabilitation access.

In conclusion, promoting equitable access to rehabilitation services requires a multifaceted approach. It is not just about ensuring physical proximity to services; it encompasses addressing socioeconomic disparities, transportation barriers, cultural factors, and the development of culturally appropriate care. Effective advocacy, community engagement, and policy changes are indispensable in achieving the goal of truly equitable access to high-quality rehabilitation care for all individuals, regardless of their background or location. Only then can we truly work towards a healthier and more equitable society.

7.5 Further Research Needs

The effectiveness of holistic rehabilitation hinges on a deeper understanding of its diverse applications across various demographics. Future research should prioritize longitudinal studies tracking patient outcomes over extended periods, comparing holistic approaches with conventional methods in controlled trials. This will provide robust evidence for the long-term benefits and cost-effectiveness of integrating these modalities. Specifically, we need more data on the effectiveness of holistic therapies in managing chronic pain conditions, a significant area where conventional treatments often fall short.

Investigating the interaction between holistic therapies and existing medication regimens is crucial. Many patients use both conventional and complementary approaches, yet the interplay between these modalities remains poorly understood. Future studies should examine potential synergistic effects, adverse interactions, and optimal sequencing of treatments. This knowledge will guide safer and more effective clinical practice.

A significant gap exists in our understanding of the cultural and socioeconomic factors that influence patient access to and engagement with holistic therapies. Research is needed to identify barriers to access—financial constraints, geographical limitations, cultural beliefs, and healthcare provider attitudes—to tailor interventions promoting equitable access across different socioeconomic strata. This includes exploring the feasibility and effectiveness of community-

based programs and telehealth initiatives.
Measuring the impact of holistic rehabilitation on quality of life requires more sophisticated assessment tools. Current measures often focus solely on functional outcomes, neglecting the important dimensions of emotional well-being, social participation, and overall life satisfaction. Development and validation of comprehensive, culturally appropriate quality-of-life measures are essential. Qualitative research methods, such as in-depth interviews and focus groups, can provide valuable insights into patients' subjective experiences and perceptions of recovery.
Furthermore, ethical considerations require ongoing research. The integration of holistic therapies raises questions about professional training, credentialing, and regulatory frameworks. Research is necessary to establish clear guidelines and standards for practice, ensuring patient safety and ethical treatment. Examining the potential for conflicts of interest, especially regarding financial incentives and practitioner biases, is vital. The development of clear ethical guidelines for research involving holistic therapies is also urgently needed.
The potential of technological advancements to support and enhance holistic rehabilitation deserves exploration. Telehealth platforms can expand access to therapies, while wearable sensors could provide objective data on patient progress and physiological responses. Research should investigate the effectiveness and safety of these technologies within holistic care models, alongside their impact on patient engagement and adherence. A key focus should be on responsible data management and patient privacy within these technologically-driven approaches.
Finally, research should delve deeper into the mechanism of action of holistic therapies. While some therapies have a demonstrated impact on physical and psychological well-being, a complete understanding of how these therapies

work is often lacking. This knowledge gap hinders the development of more targeted and precise treatments. Investing in mechanistic research is crucial to advance both the understanding and the application of holistic rehabilitation. Such an exploration would open avenues for developing better treatment protocols and training for healthcare professionals, resulting in more successful rehabilitation outcomes across the board. These are not exhaustive, but highlight key areas needing further investigation to optimize holistic rehabilitation for all patients. A collaborative effort involving healthcare professionals, researchers, and patients themselves is essential to make significant strides in this field.

www.ingramcontent.com/pod-product-compliance
Lightning Source LLC
LaVergne TN
LVHW022022200926
848481LV00007B/2493
* 9 7 9 8 3 4 8 5 5 8 2 5 3 *